The Beauty Student's
Face Makeup Charts

This book belongs to

____

____

____

____

Published by Noon Sun Handy Books
amazon.com/author/noonsun

Welcome to the world of face charts!

Are you an aspiring makeup artist? A beauty consultant in training? Or simply someone who loves experimenting with new looks for yourself and your friends? You'll find the face charts in this book an indispensable tool.

The idea is simple — and fun. Grab your beauty toolkit (blush, eyeliner, lipstick, everything!) and let your imagination loose while you give free rein to your creativity. By coloring in our face charts, you can try out different makeup combinations to find one that is uniquely "you."

Of course, you can also use these charts to come up with great looks for your beauty clients, for a model doing a photo shoot, or for a bride on her big day. Along with the facial outlines themselves, there are spaces for recording the various beauty products you used for a particular look, allowing you to recreate it in the future.

As one face chart enthusiast has observed, "It's a great way to play and explore. The more I work with the charts, the more new things I learn. One idea leads to another, and before long I've come up with a dozen or more great looks!"

A tip: If you want to see some of the amazing things people are doing with makeup and face charts, just do a web search for "face chart videos." Prepare to be amazed and inspired!

Name of Look ______________________

Evening ◯ **Daytime** ◯

Face

Moisturizer

Concealer

Foundation

Highlight/Blush

Eyes

Brows

Eyelid

Liner

Crease

Mascara

Lips

Liner

Lip Color

Gloss

Notes

Name of Look

Evening ○ Daytime ○

Face

Moisturizer

Concealer

Foundation

Highlight/Blush

Eyes

Brows

Eyelid

Liner

Crease

Mascara

Lips

Liner

Lip Color

Gloss

Notes

Name of Look ______

Evening ○ **Daytime** ○

Face

Moisturizer

Foundation

Concealer

Highlight/Blush

Eyes

Brows

Eyelid

Liner

Crease

Mascara

Lips

Liner

Lip Color

Gloss

Notes

Name of Look ______________________

Evening ○ **Daytime** ○

Face

Moisturizer

Concealer

Foundation

Highlight/Blush

Eyes

Brows

Eyelid

Liner

Crease

Mascara

Lips

Liner

Lip Color

Gloss

Notes

Name of Look ______________________

Evening ○ **Daytime** ○

Face

Moisturizer

Concealer

Foundation

Highlight/Blush

Eyes

Brows

Eyelid

Liner

Crease

Mascara

Lips

Liner

Lip Color

Gloss

Notes

Name of Look ______________________

Evening ○ **Daytime** ○

Face

Moisturizer

Concealer

Foundation

Highlight/Blush

Eyes

Brows

Eyelid

Liner

Crease

Mascara

Lips

Liner

Lip Color

Gloss

Notes

Name of Look

Evening ○ **Daytime** ○

Face

Moisturizer

Concealer

Foundation

Highlight/Blush

Eyes

Brows

Eyelid

Liner

Crease

Mascara

Lips

Liner

Lip Color

Gloss

Notes

Name of Look

Evening ◯ **Daytime** ◯

Face

Moisturizer

Concealer

Foundation

Highlight/Blush

Eyes

Brows

Eyelid

Liner

Crease

Mascara

Lips

Liner

Lip Color

Gloss

Notes

Name of Look ______________________

Evening ○ **Daytime** ○

Face

Moisturizer

Concealer

Foundation

Highlight/Blush

Eyes

Brows

Eyelid

Liner

Crease

Mascara

Lips

Liner

Lip Color

Gloss

Notes

Name of Look ______________________

Evening ○ **Daytime** ○

Face

Moisturizer

Concealer

Foundation

Highlight/Blush

Eyes

Brows

Eyelid

Liner

Crease

Mascara

Lips

Liner

Lip Color

Gloss

Notes

Name of Look ______________________

Evening ○ **Daytime** ○

Face

Moisturizer

Concealer

Foundation

Highlight/Blush

Eyes

Brows

Eyelid

Liner

Crease

Mascara

Lips

Liner

Lip Color

Gloss

Notes

Name of Look ______________________________

Evening ◯ **Daytime** ◯

Face

Moisturizer

Concealer

Foundation

Highlight/Blush

Eyes

Brows

Eyelid

Liner

Crease

Mascara

Lips

Liner

Lip Color

Gloss

Notes

Name of Look ______________________

Evening ○ **Daytime** ○

Face

Moisturizer

Concealer

Foundation

Highlight/Blush

Eyes

Brows

Eyelid

Liner

Crease

Mascara

Lips

Liner

Lip Color

Gloss

Notes

Name of Look ______________________

Evening ○ **Daytime** ○

Face

Moisturizer

Concealer

Foundation

Highlight/Blush

Eyes

Brows

Eyelid

Liner

Crease

Mascara

Lips

Liner

Lip Color

Gloss

Notes

Name of Look ______________________

Evening ○ **Daytime** ○

Face

Moisturizer

Concealer

Foundation

Highlight/Blush

Eyes

Brows

Eyelid

Liner

Crease

Mascara

Lips

Liner

Lip Color

Gloss

Notes

Name of Look ______________________

Evening ◯ **Daytime** ◯

Face

Moisturizer

Concealer

Foundation

Highlight/Blush

Eyes

Brows

Eyelid

Liner

Crease

Mascara

Lips

Liner

Lip Color

Gloss

Notes

Name of Look ______________________

Evening ○ **Daytime** ○

Face

Moisturizer

Concealer

Foundation

Highlight/Blush

Eyes

Brows

Eyelid

Liner

Crease

Mascara

Lips

Liner

Lip Color

Gloss

Notes

Name of Look ______________________

Evening ○ **Daytime** ○

Face

Moisturizer

Concealer

Foundation

Highlight/Blush

Eyes

Brows

Eyelid

Liner

Crease

Mascara

Lips

Liner

Lip Color

Gloss

Notes

Name of Look ______________________

Evening ◯ **Daytime** ◯

Face

Moisturizer

Concealer

Foundation

Highlight/Blush

Eyes

Brows

Eyelid

Liner

Crease

Mascara

Lips

Liner

Lip Color

Gloss

Notes

Name of Look ______________________

Evening ○ **Daytime** ○

Face

Moisturizer

Concealer

Foundation

Highlight/Blush

Eyes

Brows

Eyelid

Liner

Crease

Mascara

Lips

Liner

Lip Color

Gloss

Notes

Name of Look ______________________

Evening ◯ **Daytime** ◯

Face

Moisturizer

Concealer

Foundation

Highlight/Blush

Eyes

Brows

Eyelid

Liner

Crease

Mascara

Lips

Liner

Lip Color

Gloss

Notes

Name of Look

Evening ○ **Daytime** ○

Face

Moisturizer

Concealer

Foundation

Highlight/Blush

Eyes

Brows

Eyelid

Liner

Crease

Mascara

Lips

Liner

Lip Color

Gloss

Notes

Name of Look ______________________

Evening ◯ **Daytime** ◯

Face

Moisturizer

Concealer

Foundation

Highlight/Blush

Eyes

Brows

Eyelid

Liner

Crease

Mascara

Lips

Liner

Lip Color

Gloss

Notes

Name of Look

Evening ○ Daytime ○

Face

Moisturizer

Concealer

Foundation

Highlight/Blush

Eyes

Brows

Eyelid

Liner

Crease

Mascara

Lips

Liner

Lip Color

Gloss

Notes

Name of Look

Evening ○ **Daytime** ○

Face

Moisturizer

Concealer

Foundation

Highlight/Blush

Eyes

Brows

Eyelid

Liner

Crease

Mascara

Lips

Liner

Lip Color

Gloss

Notes

Name of Look ______________________

Evening ○ Daytime ○

Face

Moisturizer

Concealer

Foundation

Highlight/Blush

Eyes

Brows

Eyelid

Liner

Crease

Mascara

Lips

Liner

Lip Color

Gloss

Notes

Name of Look ______________________

Evening ○ **Daytime** ○

Face

Moisturizer

Concealer

Foundation

Highlight/Blush

Eyes

Brows

Eyelid

Liner

Crease

Mascara

Lips

Liner

Lip Color

Gloss

Notes

Name of Look ______________________

Evening ◯ **Daytime** ◯

Face

Moisturizer

Concealer

Foundation

Highlight/Blush

Eyes

Brows

Eyelid

Liner

Crease

Mascara

Lips

Liner

Lip Color

Gloss

Notes

Name of Look ______________________

Evening ○ **Daytime** ○

Face

Moisturizer

Concealer

Foundation

Highlight/Blush

Eyes

Brows

Eyelid

Liner

Crease

Mascara

Lips

Liner

Lip Color

Gloss

Notes

Name of Look ______________________

Evening ○ **Daytime** ○

Face

Moisturizer

Concealer

Foundation

Highlight/Blush

Eyes

Brows

Eyelid

Liner

Crease

Mascara

Lips

Liner

Lip Color

Gloss

Notes

Name of Look

Evening ○ **Daytime** ○

Face

Moisturizer

Concealer

Foundation

Highlight/Blush

Eyes

Brows

Eyelid

Liner

Crease

Mascara

Lips

Liner

Lip Color

Gloss

Notes

Name of Look ______________________

Evening ◯ **Daytime** ◯

Face

Moisturizer

Concealer

Foundation

Highlight/Blush

Eyes

Brows

Eyelid

Liner

Crease

Mascara

Lips

Liner

Lip Color

Gloss

Notes

Name of Look

Evening ◯ **Daytime** ◯

Face

Moisturizer

Concealer

Foundation

Highlight/Blush

Eyes

Brows

Eyelid

Liner

Crease

Mascara

Lips

Liner

Lip Color

Gloss

Notes

Name of Look ______________________

Evening ◯ **Daytime** ◯

Face

Moisturizer

Concealer

Foundation

Highlight/Blush

Eyes

Brows

Eyelid

Liner

Crease

Mascara

Lips

Liner

Lip Color

Gloss

Notes

Name of Look ______________________

Evening ◯ **Daytime** ◯

Face

Moisturizer

Concealer

Foundation

Highlight/Blush

Eyes

Brows

Eyelid

Liner

Crease

Mascara

Lips

Liner

Lip Color

Gloss

Notes

Name of Look ______________________

Evening ○ **Daytime** ○

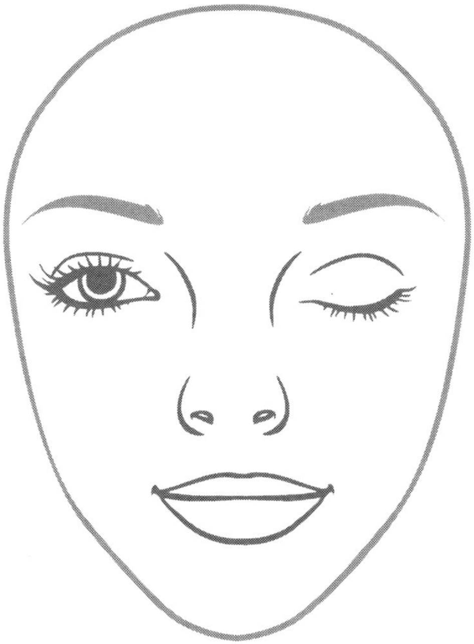

Face

Moisturizer

Foundation

Concealer

Highlight/Blush

Eyes

Brows

Eyelid

Liner

Crease

Mascara

Lips

Liner

Lip Color

Gloss

Notes

Name of Look ______________________

Evening ◯ **Daytime** ◯

Face

Moisturizer

Concealer

Foundation

Highlight/Blush

Eyes

Brows

Eyelid

Liner

Crease

Mascara

Lips

Liner

Lip Color

Gloss

Notes

Name of Look

Evening ◯ **Daytime** ◯

Face

Moisturizer

Concealer

Foundation

Highlight/Blush

Eyes

Brows

Eyelid

Liner

Crease

Mascara

Lips

Liner

Lip Color

Gloss

Notes

Name of Look ______________________

Evening ○ **Daytime** ○

Face

Moisturizer

Concealer

Foundation

Highlight/Blush

Eyes

Brows

Eyelid

Liner

Crease

Mascara

Lips

Liner

Lip Color

Gloss

Notes

Name of Look ______________________________

Evening ◯ **Daytime** ◯

Face

Moisturizer

Concealer

Foundation

Highlight/Blush

Eyes

Brows

Eyelid

Liner

Crease

Mascara

Lips

Liner

Lip Color

Gloss

Notes

Name of Look ______________________

Evening ◯ **Daytime** ◯

Face

Moisturizer

Concealer

Foundation

Highlight/Blush

Eyes

Brows

Eyelid

Liner

Crease

Mascara

Lips

Liner

Lip Color

Gloss

Notes

Name of Look ______________________

Evening ○ **Daytime** ○

Face

Moisturizer

Concealer

Foundation

Highlight/Blush

Eyes

Brows

Eyelid

Liner

Crease

Mascara

Lips

Liner

Lip Color

Gloss

Notes

Name of Look ____________________

Evening ○ **Daytime** ○

Face

Moisturizer

Concealer

Foundation

Highlight/Blush

Eyes

Brows

Eyelid

Liner

Crease

Mascara

Lips

Liner

Lip Color

Gloss

Notes

Name of Look

Evening ○ **Daytime** ○

Face

Moisturizer

Concealer

Foundation

Highlight/Blush

Eyes

Brows

Eyelid

Liner

Crease

Mascara

Lips

Liner

Lip Color

Gloss

Notes

Name of Look ______________________

Evening ○ **Daytime** ○

Face

Moisturizer

Concealer

Foundation

Highlight/Blush

Eyes

Brows

Eyelid

Liner

Crease

Mascara

Lips

Liner

Lip Color

Gloss

Notes

Name of Look ______________________

Evening ○ **Daytime** ○

Face

Moisturizer

____

Concealer

____

Foundation

____

Highlight/Blush

____

Eyes

Brows

____

Eyelid

____

Liner

____

Crease

____

Mascara

____

Lips

Liner

____

Lip Color

____

Gloss

____

Notes

Name of Look ______________________

Evening ○ **Daytime** ○

Face

Moisturizer

Concealer

Foundation

Highlight/Blush

Eyes

Brows

Eyelid

Liner

Crease

Mascara

Lips

Liner

Lip Color

Gloss

Notes

Name of Look

Evening ○ **Daytime** ○

Face

Moisturizer

Concealer

Foundation

Highlight/Blush

Eyes

Brows

Eyelid

Liner

Crease

Mascara

Lips

Liner

Lip Color

Gloss

Notes

Name of Look

Evening ◯ Daytime ◯

Face

Moisturizer

Concealer

Foundation

Highlight/Blush

Eyes

Brows

Eyelid

Liner

Crease

Mascara

Lips

Liner

Lip Color

Gloss

Notes

Name of Look ______________________

Evening ○ **Daytime** ○

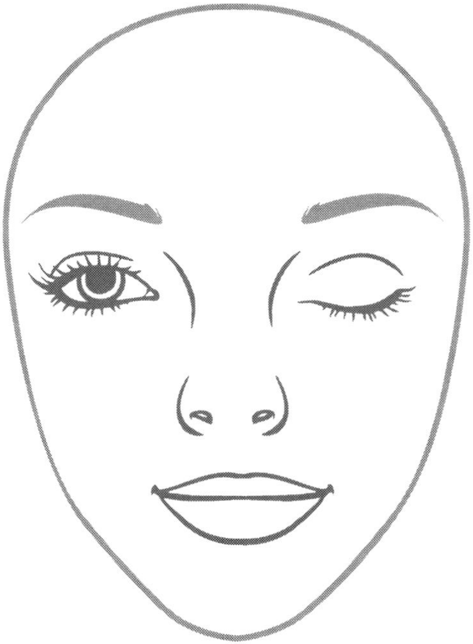

Face

Moisturizer

Foundation

Concealer

Highlight/Blush

Eyes

Brows

Eyelid

Liner

Crease

Mascara

Lips

Liner

Lip Color

Gloss

Notes

Name of Look

Evening ◯ **Daytime** ◯

Face

Moisturizer

Concealer

Foundation

Highlight/Blush

Eyes

Brows

Eyelid

Liner

Crease

Mascara

Lips

Liner

Lip Color

Gloss

Notes

Name of Look ______________________

Evening ○ **Daytime** ○

Face

Moisturizer

Concealer

Foundation

Highlight/Blush

Eyes

Brows

Eyelid

Liner

Crease

Mascara

Lips

Liner

Lip Color

Gloss

Notes

Name of Look

Evening ◯ Daytime ◯

Face

Moisturizer

Foundation

Concealer

Highlight/Blush

Eyes

Brows

Eyelid

Liner

Crease

Mascara

Lips

Liner

Lip Color

Gloss

Notes

Name of Look ______________________

Evening ○ **Daytime** ○

Face

Moisturizer

Concealer

Foundation

Highlight/Blush

Eyes

Brows

Eyelid

Liner

Crease

Mascara

Lips

Liner

Lip Color

Gloss

Notes

Name of Look ______________________

Evening ○ **Daytime** ○

Face

Moisturizer

Concealer

Foundation

Highlight/Blush

Eyes

Brows

Eyelid

Liner

Crease

Mascara

Lips

Liner

Lip Color

Gloss

Notes

Name of Look ______________________

Evening ○ **Daytime** ○

Face

Moisturizer

Concealer

Foundation

Highlight/Blush

Eyes

Brows

Eyelid

Liner

Crease

Mascara

Lips

Liner

Lip Color

Gloss

Notes

Name of Look ______________________

Evening ◯ **Daytime** ◯

Face

Moisturizer

Concealer

Foundation

Highlight/Blush

Eyes

Brows

Eyelid

Liner

Crease

Mascara

Lips

Liner

Lip Color

Gloss

Notes

Name of Look ______

Evening ○ **Daytime** ○

Face

Moisturizer

Concealer

Foundation

Highlight/Blush

Eyes

Brows

Eyelid

Liner

Crease

Mascara

Lips

Liner

Lip Color

Gloss

Notes

Name of Look ______________________

Evening ○ Daytime ○

Face

Moisturizer

Concealer

Foundation

Highlight/Blush

Eyes

Brows

Eyelid

Liner

Crease

Mascara

Lips

Liner

Lip Color

Gloss

Notes

Name of Look ____________________

Evening ○ **Daytime** ○

Face

Moisturizer

Foundation

Concealer

Highlight/Blush

Eyes

Brows

Eyelid

Liner

Crease

Mascara

Lips

Liner

Lip Color

Gloss

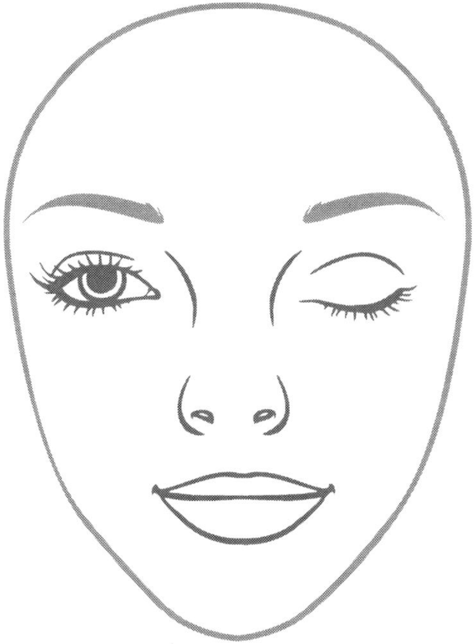

Notes

Name of Look ____________________

Evening ◯ **Daytime** ◯

Face

Moisturizer

Concealer

Foundation

Highlight/Blush

Eyes

Brows

Eyelid

Liner

Crease

Mascara

Lips

Liner

Lip Color

Gloss

Notes

Name of Look ______________________

Evening ○ **Daytime** ○

Face

Moisturizer

Concealer

Foundation

Highlight/Blush

Eyes

Brows

Eyelid

Liner

Crease

Mascara

Lips

Liner

Lip Color

Gloss

Notes

Name of Look

Evening ○ **Daytime** ○

Face

Moisturizer

Concealer

Foundation

Highlight/Blush

Eyes

Brows

Eyelid

Liner

Crease

Mascara

Lips

Liner

Lip Color

Gloss

Notes

Name of Look

Evening ◯ Daytime ◯

Face

Moisturizer

Concealer

Foundation

Highlight/Blush

Eyes

Brows

Eyelid

Liner

Crease

Mascara

Lips

Liner

Lip Color

Gloss

Notes

Made in the USA
Las Vegas, NV
12 February 2023